The Good Seed

The Good Seed

Planted with Purpose: A Growth Journey

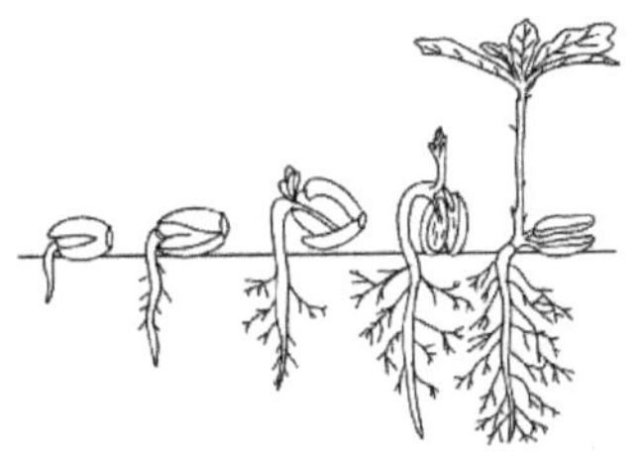

Stephany Staple

ISBN: 978-976-655-099-8

Cover Artwork By: Corianne Chambers

DEDICATION

To my beloved Great-grandmother

This book stands as a testament to the profound impact you have had on my life and the lives of countless others. My dear great-grandmother, you were more than a matriarch; you were a beacon of light, a steadfast pillar of faith, and a source of unwavering love. With your wisdom as my compass, you instilled in me the values of prayer, humility, and perseverance.

As a Pastor, you taught me the importance of connecting with something greater than myself, reminding me that true strength lies in surrendering to a higher power.

With profound gratitude and immeasurable love, I dedicate this book to you, Elfreda Staple. Your legacy lives on through these pages and me.

PREFACE

The Good Seed
Planted With Purpose: A Growth Journey
By Stephany Staple

Life is not a bed of roses, but have you ever felt that you've been given quite a thorny path to trod? Maybe life has consistently reminded you that the only thing that remains constant is change.

I want to offer you hope. Hope that you can overcome your pain and live to bear fruit; hope that temporary sufferings are just that--temporary and that perseverance can often mark the difference between a transformed trajectory and the same ol' same ol'.

I've been through countless ups and downs, tragedies that threatened to wreck my very identity. Yet I've found that when you cultivate deep roots of faith and hope, supported by positive deeds, you can overcome anything.

This book is not a "cure-all" --your circumstance is unique to you. However, I offer you some key life lessons that I believe can help you discover the strength and knowledge to persevere toward hope and, ultimately, your better, best self.

Are you ready to journey with me? Keep reading.

CONTENTS

ACKNOWLEDGMENTS

This recount of my life and the journey to wellness has been a soul cleanse for me. But there are a few people without whom my life's journey would have had several more trepidating twists and turns, people whom, if it were not for them, this beautifully liberating and honest recount would never have made it to these pages.

Firstly, I'd like to thank my aunt, Deloree Staple- for her unwavering belief in me. You have stood by me 'in thick and thin', my constant support even when the world seems to shift beneath my feet. You remind me exactly who I am and reignite my will to dream and to REACH! When life's hurdles have been stacked like an insurmountable tower, you give me the boost I've needed time and time again ---tangible and intangible to climb over and above, to REACH upward towards the goal- my sunlight. THANK YOU!

To Elfreda Staple, my dearest "Mama Freda", you laid my foundation – having raised me from the tender age of a 4-

month baby. Your lessons and example of being resilient and strong have saved me. You ingrained a strong sense of "self" and God -you gave me the moral compass I'd have needed to find my way. Your love and lessons have anchored my sails when the winds of life have blown gusty winds of doubt and threatened to throw me off course and tatter my sails. I didn't know it then, but you taught me how to survive any storm and showed me the importance of taking care of others and reaching inward to depend on and take care of myself. I will always treasure your love and sacrifice for me. Even in death, your legacy lives on through me. I promise.

I thank my dad, Andrew Staple, for doing all you did the way you knew how. I learned early on that I needed to develop a sense of self-reliance, a 'broad back' and quickly land on my own feet. Because of you – but still, you have not left me.

To Kymone Douglas, my best friend for all seasons – thank you for ALL OF IT, for walking with me through the fire and the floods of my life. To Stacia Davidson, "the Raw Boss" I think I found you; or we found each other when I needed it most. Thank you for teaching me to actively love myself through the way I eat--- you led me down the path of true physical healing. After all, we are what we eat! Although it was you, Danishka Williams, who first introduced me to the wholesomeness of eating well and to GOOD HEALTH! Thank you both for your abundant supply of resources and information, practical, delicious eating the RAW way!

Finally, I'd like to thank you, my cherished readers. Getting the story told has been deeply satisfying but to have it read & received by you, my dear readers, is an unexpected gift. I pray you find the path to healing for your body, mind, and spirit through this book and know that wherever you are on your sojourn, you can still choose to LIVE by choosing DAILY what you put into your body, what you plant into your spirit and what your mind dwells upon. They all bear fruit in their season, choose well- LIVE WELL.

Thank you from the bottom of my heart.

INTRODUCTION

Heavenly Father,

In 3 John 2, you remind us, "Beloved, I pray that you may prosper in all things and be in good health, even as your soul prospers." We know, Father, that You desire holistic health and prosperity in mind, body, and spirit.

For every reader and person who comes in contact with this manuscript of my (continuous) journey to physical, emotional, and spiritual healing, my prayer is that they will see themselves across the pages of this book; that an amplified voice is given to the inner workings and brokenness of their bodies and hearts. You have seen how they've struggled to process every trial, failure, and disappointment that has ever beset them.

I pray they will know that You see us as we bravely navigate new and uncharted waters with an uncommon smile that masks years of pain. Pain that we don't have to own, always. And that the holder of this book, this promising sojourner of life, will feel total freedom to feel, grow and heal as we process together. May they enter into this journey expecting hope, realizing that there is more than just a silver lining to their experiences but a promise, with their name on it, that they can claim so that they may prosper in all things *and be in good health, even as their soul prospers.*

May good seeds be planted in their soil while weeds continue to be uprooted with force. May we look back at the end of this journey and joyfully acknowledge that we have not only grown but blossomed. May they grow in purpose, direction, and wisdom, allowing positive change to overtake them while opening themself to the lessons of the rain.

May they be reminded that they are the good seed, and may they live to reap the bountiful harvest You desire for them, the harvest that allows them to live purposefully and to plant good seeds in the lives of others around them.

May they bloom and prosper in all things now and always. May they bloom and prosper in accordance with Your word.

Amen

CHAPTER ONE

A Bad Seed

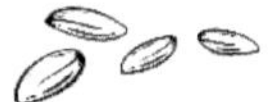

PLANTED FOR PURPOSE

Who determines the quality of a seed? I suppose the clear answer is the farmer…but what happens when the farmer plants a bad seed and that seed starts to take root? What happens when that bad seed is planted in you?

The impact of a bad seed planted early can often make growth quite difficult, especially when its soil is *the mind.* Growing up, I had feelings of pain, rejection, and loneliness planted by farmers that perhaps could do no better. I was fortunate, though, to also have good farmers consistently plant good seeds of purpose in me. It would be up to me to decide which seeds I'd allow to take root. It was never going to be an easy choice. It would actually turn out to be a *battle of the minds,* but it is often in the struggle that the most resilient seeds fight to survive to birth the strongest plants. I am that plant.

I had the pleasure of living with my great-grandmother throughout my childhood. Being the pastor that she was, she raised me with a firm and Godly hand, strong in her convictions, all the while oozing a heart of pure gold. I loved this woman with all of me. She made sure I knew my daily routine: school, church, back home, then repeat. There was no wavering, of course--not under her watch. You'd fall weary searching for a woman who could have mothered me as she did. She threw herself into the role from when I was about four (4) months young, rooting me firmly in a faith that would carry me through some of life's darkest times.

I'm not sure how else I would have coped with the news that I had just been diagnosed with PCOS at the tender age of 17 years. I remember how cold the doctor's office was. She had just taken a few samples from me after hearing me reel off the growing list of *weird things I had noticed* about my period at the time. In almost a flash, she had disappeared to a room nearby. She took what I thought could have been a day and a half to return. While I sat there, I couldn't help but think about how *helpless* and *clueless* I felt.

I was only 17 and had already grown into an undeniable sense of independence in my short life, yet, at that moment I felt empty and aimless. I remembered how I had tried ignoring, no, more like stuffing down, all the symptoms I had throughout 5th form, crying in the shower when the pain was unbearable. Nothing seemed to work, not even the "dog blood bush" my great-grandmother recommended. I wondered about my future. So many--my great-grandmother and aunt especially--saw endless possibilities for me. Still, I often yearned to get even half of the vision that they had. My young eyes had been so dimmed by pain that my eyes remained blurry. Before then, I had a troubling feeling that something was…*off*…I'd have long stretches without my period, only for it to return with a vengeance about twice in another month. If that crazy cycle wasn't enough, I had to deal with my conflicting teenage emotions bubbling up inside me, wanting to find somewhere to escape.

I remember one Sports Day before I was diagnosed. I was panicked--I hadn't seen my period for a good while now, so after spending a considerable amount of time reflecting, I couldn't hold it in any longer. I decided to tell my dad. Little did I know, I was signing my own "stay at home" card, as that was the very instruction I was given. I could have erupted with the frustration I felt that day--I got no answer for the reason *and* had to miss out on probably the most fun I'd have all school year. It did leave a lesson with me, though--support wasn't going to be easy to come by when things were this uncertain.

"What was taking this doctor so long?" My reflections as I waited were punctuated by interrupting worries that she'd come back with a diagnosis I wasn't ready for. Then, footsteps and my chart found their way through the door. "Your symptoms indicate that you have something called *Polycystic Ovary Syndrome (PCOS)*." I have never drawn so many blanks in my mind all at once. I waited for her to continue, "This means you'll have to start taking birth control." I drifted into space for one more minute, then saw myself nod, thank her, then leave. She might as well have told me I had one more year to live. I'm not sure I would have known the difference. I allowed her life sentence to flow freely out of my left ear. "Life may need to change, but not now," I decided.

Growing up, I didn't always have my *ducks in a row*. I screamed for attention, especially my father's--committing the casual teenage offense here and there, ruffling a few of his feathers. While the exact purpose of my misdemeanors may have been blurry to those around me, my mind was committed to the task. My mind knew what my heart wanted: to be the apple of my father's eye or *even just one of them*. It's probably every girl's dream, and I was no different. Common sense should have told me that while I'd get even a fraction of the attention I longed for with my antics, our bonding process needed a much more than just these intermittent run-ins. Night after night, I would sit up in the lonely darkness of my room, finding that I was being hit in the face by seeds of unworthiness. These seeds sprouted feelings of resentment and rejection in me. It grew so strongly and stubbornly in my heart that I fought with my entire being to outrun it--until one day when my heart finally caught up with my legs.

Like teenage girls often do, I had a serious crush—only it was a unique type of crush; picture your typical teenage drama – "*situationship*" that your daddy doesn't want to hear one more thing about; yeah, *that kind*…but that gave me just enough of a spark to add fuel to the fire that was raging within my 15-year-old heart. Over time, I had learned to find small cracks in my great-grandmother's school-church-home routine, so I pursued this juvenile bond with every rebellious fiber of my being; but my dad wouldn't have it. Every warning he threw my way gave me added resolve to keep pursuing it. I finally had the consistent talks, concern, and attention I desired. I was still missing his approval, of course, but I told myself that was a necessary compromise for the benefits achieved. I had to find a way to propel it even further. I could almost see the light bulb being switched on in my brain when

I realized I had to run away. I ran so far *(not that far actually)* I ended up by my grand aunt's house, reveling in even a few ounces of accomplishment that I had fulfilled my goal. My dad was livid, but his presence was guaranteed. I felt like I had gained even a small victory. He was concerned, he *cared* even…*and yet, I heard--almost as clear as day-- "You're looking for love in all the wrong places, Stephany."* I could run, I could hide, I could even rebel…but I couldn't outrun God or my nagging conscience.

What was wrong with me? Despite the overwhelming emptiness that would sometimes try to cloak my heart space, I had my fair share of cheerleaders. Along with my great-grandmother ("Mama"), I had an amazing aunt who remains one of my most ardent supporters to this day, a woman who not only talked the talk but truly walked the walk in all the ways that mattered. When I tell you that this woman paid for *all* my education, from high school to college, always encouraging me all the while having her own family…she had even traveled miles to ensure I secured my space, was registered, and prepared with the tools for my college years. Sometimes I truly believe that God uses humans as physical extensions of His loving arms to remind us that He never truly leaves us or forsakes us. Without her love, provision, and added nurturing, I'm not sure how my roots would eventually find their way to pulling the mineral from the soil. I knew I was blessed…but at nights, when my head would hit my pillow, I'd be alone again…alone to face myself…alone to come to grips with any residual feelings of lost love that I craved—after all why didn't my father do that?

When I ran away, it was as if I was bursting with pent-up emotions, and my heart almost immediately shot up through my chest and threatened to escape my wide-open jaws, desperately gasping for air. It's a frightening thing to suddenly come to the realization, mid-rebellion, that you have absolutely no idea what it is that you're *really* doing. I could have been scooped up and never seen again. I could have become a statistic…but in the heat of the moment, neither of those nor any other remotely dangerous possibilities were coming anywhere close to my mind. I just knew that I had run into what I wanted to be the last "head-butting" argument with my dad. He put his foot down for what seemed like the *millionth* time about this boy, and it was as though he had finally squeezed the trigger to unlock my wild, chaotic, helpless, hopelessly *hopeful* emotions. Oh, I was full of so much hope that I'd be able to escape myself, his opposition, and all negative consequences. I was so lost, and yet, I truly believe that this may actually have been the start of my *awakening*.

My uncle (who was more like a dad to me) flung me straight into counseling. It wasn't quite the attention I was looking for, but I was refreshed to finally have an outlet where I could release some of the darkness that was pent up so deep inside me.

The sessions helped, well, at least for giving me some perspective. I didn't have all I wanted in the emotional support I needed, but I started to awaken to the fact that despite the bad, so much good had been planted in me. Amongst the many seeds, I could choose to water the good seed in me. Even after the first stage of overcoming it, though, I'd have soon realized

that my journey *as the good seed* had only just begun. If you think

about the life of a seed, it's just when the seed believes it is

ready to see the first light that it must then die.

CHAPTER 2
The Seed Must Die

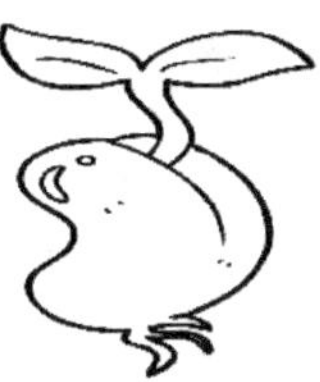

A seed must first die for it to experience transformation… transformation into destiny, into purpose. Likewise, we experience death on many levels, moments that bring us to our knees and rock the world around us, but from these tragedies come the birthing of unexpected new beginnings.

What was I running from? Myself, maybe. Every now and then, I was haunted by the doctor's diagnosis echoing loudly in my head from time to time, with the words "P-C-O-S" and "birth control" ringing repeatedly. My lonely wilderness only seemed to grow as I drowned my worries in a sea of pulsating parties. I mindlessly consumed random junk food like I didn't receive a life-altering diagnosis a few years prior. I traded my health for temporary fixes of pleasure, hoping, perhaps, that they would help me preserve some sense of "self" --something that seemed to be slipping further and further outside of my grasp with every thought of my new fate.

"What if I can't have children?" "Why was I always in so much pain?" "What was happening inside me?" I didn't dare ask aloud, and strangely—or not, the former more than the latter thought tore away at the hopes I had always carried of having a family of my own one day in the future. How *is* a teenager *supposed* to cope with something like this? I didn't know what I needed at the time. I felt like I was lost at sea and without a possible clue. Google wasn't even a "thing" for me back then. I barely had access to any technology, so finding out more about my condition on my own was unbelievably difficult. I had no one to *share notes* with, or to tell me that what I was going through was symptoms associated with PCOS. I just knew that *Bio class* had never featured anyone with a period lasting an entire week or resulting in fainting spells.

Looking back, I wish I had people around me with the experience to guide me on this, with a lot of good information and the right, welcoming, friendly approach to quell my fears and steady my decisions. Instead, I was hampered by the self-imposed burden of not wanting to weigh down the people close to me with my heavy load. So, for a long time, I told no one.

I knew they meant well, but I couldn't bring myself to let them know what I was dealing with--or *avoiding,* for that matter. After all, they couldn't really change my situation —at least, I didn't think so.

I had a best friend though, Kymone, who gave meaning to the saying, *"Good fren better dan pocket money,"* as we say here in Jamaica [meaning -- Good friends are better to have than even cash in an emergency]. Even without a dollar to my name, this girl was my *ride-or-die* before I ever knew that was a "thing." I had no idea exactly how profoundly her presence would impact my life. ***Proverbs 17:17 says, "A friend loves at all times, and a brother [or sister] is born for a time of*** *adversity."* We often think of friends like the ones we want to enjoy the best of times with, the ones who share in your highs and celebrate you. However, I've come to learn that a true friend is "born" for the *lows* of your life as well. In fact, that is truly when you know…who's in your corner or valley, as the case might be. It's not up to you to *keep* them from being *too burdened* by your burdens. Being there for you in times like those is not only what tests the *mettle* and measure of your friendship, but it gives them the opportunity to spring into action on your behalf, fulfilling their God-given purpose in your life to divide sorrow. I can humbly and confidently say this is the measure of my friend Kymone.

I remember the day like it was just yesterday--I was on step one of my daily routines. A 22-year-old college student now, I had started "coming into my own," discovering the joy of navigating school life *(life overall)* with my best friend, Kymone. Have you ever felt like you knew someone from way back, even though you just met them? Well, from the beginning, that was Kymone and I. To borrow from my

Jamaican parlance *"batty an' bench,"* you could say when you see her, you see me and *(well, you know the rest!)*. But more than that, her support would become so real in due time.

The day was normal enough--I was up, bright and early, ready to take on the new challenges of taking care of my rock-hardy great-grandmother--my anchor, my strong tree. It had been like this for the past seven years. I had become her primary caregiver, although she would only allow me to do so much. This woman, who taught me most of everything I know, including to pray about everything, from the life-changing matters to the lowly headache, was now fading—and no prayers seemed to change that.

Alzheimer's took so many parts of her; her memory, her personality, her confidence; but never the word of God, which seemed deeply rooted in her. She was such a strong, formidable woman. I watched her sing at her own son's funeral without surrendering a tear. She'd go on to repeat this enduring resolve as she buried several other relatives with a dry face that, somehow, still shone with the radiance of a woman confident that she would one day be reunited with them in Heaven. She kept a lot in, and at this point, her mind became even more of a *pandora's box* of sorts, with all her reflections, pain, and secrets now managing to elude her. She was always able to find her faith, though. Giving up her pastor's seat, she lay herself at the foot of the cross, clinging firmly to her God in breathtaking fashion.

Even in her sickness, she was something to behold. I'd help with cooking, cleaning, clothes washing, and the Sunday Bible reading, but this woman, my "Mama," saw sickness as the enemy of her freedom. I remember having to literally nail the doors shut when I'd leave for school because there was not an open door that did not present itself as an invitation to take a good walk to only God knows where--because she surely wouldn't.

With my feelings of isolation growing, I started wondering how common it was for a 14-year-old 8th grader [as I was when this began] to have had the role of primary caregiver for their great-grandmother or any other family member for that matter. Yet then again, my life was never what I thought to be typical--I wasn't raised by or with my mother and my father, who lived *nearby* rather than with me. Perhaps, though, I was restricted to the limitations of my perception of my own reality because I was flabbergasted to know that my dad, for example, saw my trading roles with Mama as a caregiver as the *natural* course of "how things should be." "After all," he'd say, "she has taken care of you, so now it is time for you to take care of her." However, I struggled to make sense of this in my teenage consciousness. I was and will forever be grateful for the incomparable sacrifices of my great-grandmother and even the privilege of loving her in service. I just wished, at the time, that someone would have seen and heard my desperate cries for an extra helping hand. I was all alone in this, yet again.

From time to time, I'd have offerings of sympathy extended to me by the kind residents of my community. I feel as though they saw my struggle to not only care for Mama, but to remain *on the straight and narrow*. The love for Mama was something that everyone felt, far and wide. There is one particular encounter that has stuck with me to this day. It involves a gentleman that I had never met before but who was clearly a congregant of my Mama Freda, stopping me mid-walk with a burning observation to get off his chest. "A wah dat yuh have on?" he blurted out. I figured it would be better for me to bite my tongue. Of course, he went on to observe that my conduct and appearance at the time were far from in keeping with the righteous standards beautifully set by Mama. It was moments like those that helped steer me back onto the right course. I certainly didn't feel it at the time, but those consistent corrections and "rebuke" turned my eyes back to Mama and what she would have expected of me. I was never living for *only myself,* and I was slowly adjusting to the thought that that would be okay.

A few years after my first PCOS diagnosis, I found myself at Knox College. I was trudging the usual throes of yet another challenging school day when I got the call. Early that morning, I did my usual, making Mama something for breakfast, but she wasn't her usual self. She didn't take it. I think I felt my heart sink to my stomach. She hadn't been her "regular self" for quite a while now, but this, …this felt different. I told her I'd be heading out, and she gave me a sweet yet telling "Goodbye." Despite my discomfort, I couldn't have known for certain that that would have been our very last earthly exchange. Hours later, I received the chilling phone call from my cousin—the unthinkable had happened. She managed to break the devastating news of my grandmother's passing and further that undertakers were awaiting me at our house. I rushed home, my heart in my hand. I almost passed out when I saw that the undertakers had not moved her and were waiting for me to return to carry her away. My Mama, my safety net, my love, my everything—gone.

I think I felt it more deeply than I allowed myself to show then; that trait of my Mama seems to have transcended to me. I couldn't afford to break into the ten million tiny pieces my heart seemed to shatter into. It wasn't quitting time yet; Mama's funeral would need to be fitting. I had learned from the best how to hold my head down and get things done amidst unspeakable pain and loss. I was no stranger to loss; even at the tender age of 5, I was able to absorb a deep sense of loss when my great-grandfather passed.

I held my tears until the day of Mama's ceremony when all floodgates burst, and I could hold it no longer. My tears flowed freely until their streaks had stained my cheeks, like buckets of water from inside my heart drowning me. Where would I go from here?

The road before me seemed to intersect and loop endlessly until it became a daunting roller coaster. I spent a considerable amount of time just struggling to find which way was true north. Still, Mama's words, her teachings, and her discipline would never be allowed to go in vain. I had rebelled and disappointed in several ways, but now… now was the time for me to honor Mama. I had no choice in the matter. My love for her would never be locked in a grave. I started unto a new path…a path that would include a complete overhaul of my daily habits and lifestyle. I put a pause on the pointless parties;

my diet got a makeover, and I zoned into my education. I was ready for the next phase, for lasting change…finally.

"Where, oh death, is your sting?" I'm thankful for this comfort, though, for it is in her death that I soon found the will to steady my roots and spring to life.

When old habits start to die, it's time for the seed to start shooting above ground, breathing in the new, fresh air, announcing life, announcing purpose.

CHAPTER 3
Shooting Above Ground

LIFE BEGINS TO SPRING FORTH

Throughout my "death journey," my roots grew so much deeper and stronger than before. It was now time for new life to start shooting above ground. A new journey was about to be unearthed.

It's easy to wonder why we are placed in less-than-favorable situations--why our parents are a *certain way* instead of our "ideal" ...why our siblings seem to get the bond, the attention, the *everything* we had longed for...why our bodies start to betray us... I didn't have solid answers to any or all of these questions, but I knew this-- I had to get a grip on my life, and with *immediate* effect. My anchor...my rock, was no longer with me, so I had no time to wallow in self-pity and sorrow. I absorbed the minerals from the soil she had placed me in, with the watering from my aunt, and began the uncomfortable, self-reinventing task of growth…it was either that or die too. Life is a constant flow; we don't get to sit still. We're either progressing or regressing, growing or shriveling, living or dying—but we are the ones who decide the quality of that experience.

In fact, I've come to the blissfully ironic realization that these strained relationships, these struggles, and seeming misfortunes, are far from chaotic coincidences. They have the potential to strengthen or weaken you, to birth purpose within you, to pressure deeply hidden treasure within you to surface. I now understood that if I were to go forward, I would have to choose my direction and push above the ground; *own my struggle, understand it,* call it what it is, and use it to propel me upward toward the sunlight, seeking out solutions, one step, one question, one connection, one change at a time. No one else could do that for me, just like no one else can grow for you…and life wasn't going to be easier.

There will always be something or someone we cannot control. But we can control ourselves and our response, and that is where our greatest energy is best focused.

I had a vision and knew I needed to pursue it. I returned to school and began getting serious about furthering my education. Still, my lifestyle changes took a little longer to get completely on board. Some things were harder to let go of entirely. I eventually visited what would only have been my second doctor about my PCOS symptoms. She assessed that the symptoms were sprouting from a hormone imbalance and recommended a pelvic ultrasound. I was hungry for information, so I opened the diagnosis letter before handing it over. I still didn't understand what PCOS was...medication was prescribed, including one that was a diabetic drug (Metformin), and Diane 5. It seemed I had more information and more solutions, but I still wasn't where I wanted to be. My food and other choices hadn't changed in a material way just yet.

I recall my sweet Aunty Deloree being the first person to present me with my first $1000 note. She would give me incentives from time to time, and I would save them and put them towards sanitary products. Sanitary products were my number 1 investment. It was almost as though my life now depended on it…but it was my life. I was determined to take responsibility, however gradual my changes had to be.

I was at least in college again, struggling my way through the sometimes-rigorous agricultural practicals at CASE, College of Agriculture, Science & Education. My period was not playing dead in even the slightest way. I'd experienced tummy pains from the week before its arrival, and they got unimaginably severe and intense on the day when my menses was about to start. Pain and tenderness in my breasts, liquid discharge, dark patches under my breasts, and increased facial hair were some of the less-than-pleasant symptoms I would eventually realize were all associated with PCOS.

I don't think I've ever truly recognized the love that my dad has for me. It's not the "princess and fairy tales" kind of love, but that he loves me is undeniable. I remember the day I got my period. Now, every pre-teen expects to get the "Period

101" lesson from their mom, right? Who else has that expertise, that nurturing touch, those understanding words? I was no stranger to that longing, but I had to hang up that expectation and cling to the reality that my mom wasn't with me to hold my hand. I'd been told that she had me while a child herself, doing what she thought best, giving me to my great-grandmother while she attempted to gain even some semblance of an education. On seeing me grappling with my first set of cramps and discomfort, my dad was the one who walked me through how to open and position my first sanitary napkin. Funnily enough, this moment just seemed like the regular course of things for me at the time, but now that I'm grown and looking back, I see where it ingrained a love within me for my dad that defies life itself. He took on much more than most fathers I knew were required to. But having been raised by Mama Freda too, we shared a common direction, and he was as consistent as he understood in caring for my needs. I loved him then, and for all its worth, I love him now.

My cheerleading duo of my aunt and Kymone, the

bestie, helped buffer my journey even more. I always felt a nagging need, to keep them unburdened which actually kept me from spilling the full details of what was going on with me. At this point, I had fainted at CASE about three times - once in the bathroom, once on the farm mid-practical, and then in my own room at home. I'd black out because of the excessive blood loss that came with my monthly periods. After a while, I was unable to go to farming practicals whenever I was on my period. I was going through four to five pads a day for the first two to three days each time. Sometimes, the pain would last right through the five days and, more frequently, a week. I wasn't sure how much longer I could continue like this. My heart longed for a possible "light at the end of the tunnel," but at the time, it just seemed like the light was very far off in the distance.

It's commonly said that "Ignorance is bliss." However, my ignorance, I think, helped to extend my suffering for much longer than it ever needed to be. I struggled to find information about *best practices* for someone who was in my shoes at the time. PCOS was still a very newly researched condition, so I was pretty much swimming upstream for the initial stages after my diagnosis. My diet, in particular, remained unchanged. I continued to enjoy processed foods and every kind of "junk" imaginable, hopelessly unaware of the connection between what went into my body and what it produced as a result.

It would also take a few years for me to fully appreciate the revelation that friends and family who care should form part of my *inner circle*…my strong support system who would go out of their way to weather any storm with me. These were "my people," yet, I chose to withhold a very important part of myself from them. I had to wrap my arms around the truth that the people who cared had demonstrated, time after time, that they were in life with me for the long haul and were worthy of being confided in. I look back and wonder how much more support and resources I could have unlocked had I let my aunt and bestie know the source of my pain.

When I shared it with my *team*, I'd learn that my aunt was actually experiencing similar struggles and could at least have been a shoulder to lean on or a lap to cry in. To tell you that she was beside herself when I finally told her would be to undermine the depth of her shock and bewilderment at my secrecy. My bestie, Kymone, probably always had a feeling without actually knowing what my condition was. I still have the jacket she gave me on one of my "off" days, and I'll always treasure it. My team helped buffer the emotional blows I'd sometimes get from remarks about my ever-changing body. One of my least favorite PCOS-related features, perhaps the bane of most women's existence--was the protruding belly. I perhaps can't count on just one hand how many times a stranger has either extended me "Congratulations" or enquired about something related to the due date of my pregnancy, to which I started practicing a brief dismissal and body language indicating I'm ready to move on from the topic.

My self-confidence took serious hits. Often, I found myself pandering to the "thief of all joy," comparison. I weighed myself against my slimmer friends, wondering if it would ever be possible for me to attain the same, or at least a similar, physical structure. I honestly just wanted this belly gone! *Is that too much to ask?* My PCOS surely thought so.

To add to my frazzled self-image, I also found myself processing my then-boyfriend's sudden decision to call "us" *quits*. I'm usually very alert, but this one threw me for a serious loop when it ended. This was the same man who helped me finance my visits to gynecologists as needed. I had confided in him about my condition, and then, like the worst kind of magic, he just decided he didn't want to be in a relationship. We spoke so well up to the day he said he wanted to call it quits. I suppose that didn't help my confidence in sharing my woes with people I thought I could trust. But I reminded myself life wasn't going to get easier; I just needed to keep getting stronger. PUSH TOWARDS THE LIGHT.

I was meant to be a resilient seed. The rain was pouring in my garden, threatening to flood and wash away every positive step I had now taken. I started comforting myself with alcohol; he was my first...and the first person who I felt truly understood me. I was devastated, but my roots of faith...my roots of perseverance…held firm, and I was anchored. I later came to understand that he was having life troubles, including some serious family issues. He felt pressured by his parents to go to school while holding down a stressful job. I can imagine how much he may have bottled up his struggles. He was never much of a talker, but I was able to bridge the communication gap through his sister, who eventually helped me "fill in the blanks."

I was still wrestling with my mind, constantly worrying if and when I would finally be better. Whenever I tried even a few changes, I'd drive myself into disillusion because I wasn't seeing the results quickly. I remember not wanting to go out because of the insensitive remarks about my weight gain... to avoid the negativity. It was at low points like these that sweet memories of Mama would come like the melody of a songbird, to my mind. I'd journey back to having to wait hours and hours for Mama to cook dinner after church. I had to attend church with her every day until the hungry wait became too much to bear.

Even memories like these somehow brought the broadest smile to my face. Any memory of Mama would do this, because, with it, I'd also be reminded to pray to talk openly with God about *everything*, including my day-to-day trials and tribulations. Time after time, I'd find myself crying out to God, "If you allow me to feel better, I'll live a better life," and I'd get a peace that I can't quite describe.

My transformation journey had only just begun. There was still a lot of letting go that needed to happen. If there is one thing true about growth, it's that it takes time--add to that patience and consistency, and then despite your falling over and over again, you're on your way to being ready for the next chapter...

CHAPTER 4
Turning A New Leaf

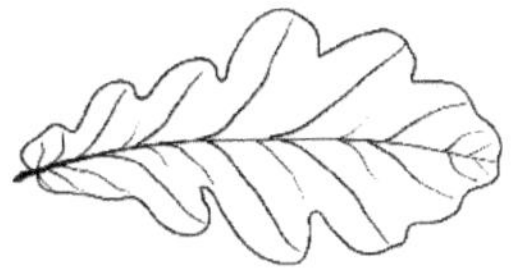

TIME FOR A FRESH START

Sometimes growth requires shedding...leaving in the past the things that deprived us of the life-giving light of hope. It takes perseverance to read past the close of the tragic chapters of your life, courage to turn the page at the risk of facing more of the same--but turn we must, to a new leaf, for the whole story has not yet been read.

So much time had passed since my first and then second diagnosis. I had started taking small steps in the right direction, but there were still a few pieces to my puzzle that I couldn't find. I knew within my heart of hearts that I needed family...I needed *community*--people who could not only relate to all that I had been through...people who could go a step further to actually provide solid resources that could pull me out of my "pit." I needed options…options that worked consistently, options that didn't confine me to a box of "must-dos". I needed something that could help show me how to take charge of my own lifestyle rather than leave me dependent on *meds* for the rest of my life. I needed something different, something new.

The year 2018 brought almost immediate highs and lows, though. I got another health blow, being diagnosed with a fibroid, but as is often true, with every dark cloud comes a silver lining if you look close enough. And as I began learning to look for it, the silver lining didn't take too long to reveal itself. I met a doctor who finally pointed me in a new direction. He defied the pill-pushing mindset that had been shoved my way by doctor after doctor, delving deeper to help me identify the *root* of my problem: my diet. It's not hard to appreciate that "garbage in" really does equate to "garbage out." Still, it isn't always easy when it comes to *internalizing* and *adjusting* to a principle like that. It certainly wasn't for me.

Over the years, I think I grew an *attachment* to the "fast and convenient" lifestyle. Any other alternative would have taken far too many resources and far too much time to prepare on a consistent basis. It didn't help that I had little to no knowledge about the *raw diet community* and their lifestyle when I first received my diagnosis.

I was seemingly in the perfect environment for it, though--like I had actually been set up for success--when I took the move to Portland to pursue agricultural studies at CASE. Agriculture had always been my strongest suit. I thought nothing much of it while studying in high school. After all, it was not a "corporate career subject," ...*you know,* one of those that will get you the high-paying job and corporate-ladder-climbing potential. My life and purpose had come full circle. This girl, who doubted herself and couldn't even dream of life beyond the there and then, has now become a beacon for small farming, singing its praises and reaping the life-changing benefits all at the same time.

I've changed from the inside out, no longer plagued by

PCOS on one of my ovaries. It has both shrunk and stopped growing. I'm no longer feeling pain from that! And can I tell you? My body figure ain't complaining either, hunnay! Remember that "pregnant looking" belly that would attract negative attention? Well, I'm pleased to report that it's no longer protruding as much. I'm no longer asked, "When are you due?" You're looking at a loss of 43 lbs./12 inches off my waist! My acne doesn't visit quite as often, and I'm more energized all around.

Again, I must praise my aunt, who counseled me when I had failed one of my CXCs--yes, one of the same ones she had paid for so generously. She looked me straight in the eyes and let me know that even the best of the best would experience failure and that I should not allow it to define me. These are the good seeds that had taken root in my life, allowing me to shoot above ground with life and start turning my new leaf. It's only fitting that the leaves play such a primary role in creating food to sustain the plant. This is what my aunt now encouraged me to do--to plant what I needed in my own space, not to despise small beginnings, to return to my roots. Imagine someone driving all the way to Portland, from Clarendon, on your behalf…to hand off your college application to the school even without your ever asking or knowing. This…*this* was and is the make and measure of my aunt, love in action…over and over and over again.

I've been blessed with a mental *load-off*. I'm no longer quite as stressed. and I enjoy a confidence that has managed to bloom both beautifully and defiantly. Moreover, I've developed a strong faith and trust in God. I know that the foundation Mama Freda built was the driving force for this one.

"There's nothing like an idea whose time has come." Indeed, I have found this to be true because it was almost serendipitous how I suddenly started to see all things falling into place to boost my success. I cut off unhelpful lifestyle habits, started receiving encouragement from my aunt to farm, got accepted to agriculture school at CASE; and funnily enough, the upward sequence of events didn't even stop there.

Soon after all this, I had the pleasure of meeting Dr. Shelly-Ann Weeks, who gave me another strong push to change my diet. It was as though I had finally started accepting God's purpose for my life, finding the sunlight. When I started to respond to the invitation to move forward with purpose, all the support I needed just started to come rushing at me with a welcoming wave.

The final light bulb got switched on a relatively normal day of scrolling through Instagram--*the millennial's sometimes mindlessly addictive "go-to" activity,* but this day was different. This was the day that my destiny would finally receive the boost it needed. **@realplantbabe – Danishka Williams** was radiant, positive, healthy, and so full of life. She shined like a radiant light, and I knew one thing: I wanted to embody the same kind of vibrancy that she did. I needed to discover her secret…what was fueling her zeal for life and for helping others. Her description painted a colorful picture of a "plant-based health coach" and "recipe creator," extending a warm invitation, "Let me help you lead a healthier, happier life."

What more could a girl like me want? After all that, I had been through, all that I had fought and grown through, and all that I had learned through, I was ready to turn a new leaf to begin writing my life's chapter of *happiness.*

At first, I had to do the *dirty work.* I had to actually *convince* myself that I was fully deserving and capable of a change like this. You know, the mind has a funny way of clinging to and even romanticizing the past--even the traumatic parts. We often find it difficult to let go, to surrender to freedom, and to change. Still, suppose we are truly serious about being transformed. In that case, we must come into a place where we are able to appreciate the lessons of the past without sacrificing and even delaying our progress into the path that is before us in the present and future. Our future selves demand it of us!

I learned, too, that my process of letting go of the past and stepping into my purpose was not going to happen overnight. I would need to release the desire for a "zip-zap-quick-fix" transformation, learning to celebrate every "small step," every "small milestone," every *slight turn in the right direction*; for without one step, without one milestone, without even an inch-turn, I would be fixed to the spot of my wounds. Small progress would indeed be counted as *progress, the best part of my process.*

I would then need to start the process of forgiving myself--forgiving my intermittent indiscretions: the *cheat day that cheated the cheat day before,* the lack of motivation from time to time, the overwhelm at taking on a whole new life change! My transformation would prove that *consistency is the key to success.*

My final lesson would manifest itself in having a *true community*--one that would serve as a source of encouragement, motivation, and accountability. This has probably been the most difficult lesson for me to learn over the years. You already know that I am "Miss Independent" --the one who doesn't like to burden her best friend, her aunt, and even her great-grandmother with the very real, very painful struggles that had burdened her body, her mind, and her soul; so, you'd know then, that reaching out to people were not automatic. I've always kept my circle close and intimate, and even those *privileged few* could not invade the space of my mind… "What had this brought me?" I started wondering to myself. I had learned to be strong, self-sufficient, and very sure of myself…but after a while spent suffering alone, your need for connection, for even a listening ear and a caring word, starts to grow. Mine was growing like a fierce weed at this point!

I encountered two amazing lifestyle coaches in Danishka Williams and, eventually, Stacia Davidson, the "Raw Boss," as we call her, **@rawfoodchallengeja**. These women would help reset my eating habits and self-limiting belief habits and overall helped me take responsibility for my self-care and holistic recovery, mind, body, and spirit. They were like lifestyle superheroes coming in to save the day and introducing me to a "Justice League" of other holistic lifestyle coaches and "doers"! I discovered that support is closer than you think and that it makes a huge difference in your recovery journey, helping you turn a fresh, new leaf. I thought my life as it was,

was pretty much how it was always going to be--but my diagnosis, my pain, was never meant to be the end, but rather the beginning of my purpose. The good seed was growing and was about to bear fruit.

CHAPTER 5
Bearing Fruit

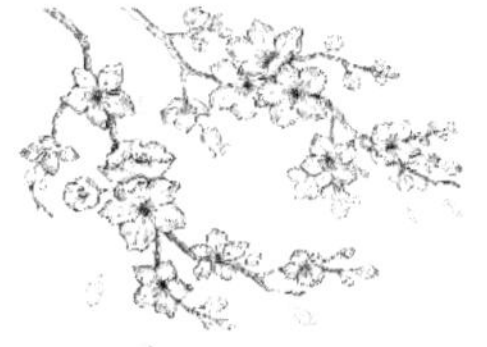

THE GOOD SEED BLOOMS

When I was young, If I had looked into the future, I would never have been able to predict my growth, my blossoming. It's amazing sometimes how limited our vision can be when all we can see is our problems. When our life view is hope-driven, we are forced to look above and beyond what we currently see, envisioning and receiving wholeheartedly the vision for success that lies ahead of us. It is at this moment that we can't help but bear fruit.

Speaking of fruits…*can I tell you?* I've been eating quite a few! Remember this girl who couldn't shake the junk food jitters, and stop partying and drinking despite diagnosis after diagnosis? I sometimes catch myself staring into the mirror and marveling at my transformation. I can now say with pure honesty and confidence that a fruit bowl or a smoothie are my go-to breakfast choices, and I have an amazing, supportive community to thank for it.

I joined the Raw Food Challenge community in June 2021. I had grown tired of being stopped by a random person, asking when the baby was due. I needed my confidence back! Imagine my disappointment when my anxiety didn't convert my diet and exercise habit changes to overnight results. I nearly lost my marbles. I was so desperate for change that I let myself think that the baggage I had taken years to accumulate would vanish away in the space of a few weeks or so. I was tempted to throw in the towel, but this time, I just wasn't alone in my own judgments and volition. Every time I picked up the phone, I'd read yet another progress report from a community member that had started their journey before me. I was able to visualize and establish my own personal goal. I was able to regenerate a hope that was deep and lasting--hope that change would eventually happen, even if not right now.

This shift in mindset would prove to be the most significant change of them all for me. Weeks passed, then months, and then another…and then one morning, while getting dressed, I found myself taking a second glance at the image that smiled back at me. My hands found themselves hugging my precious belly, almost looking for the extra bulge that had taken up residence there for such a long time. My heart must have skipped even half a beat when I realized my bloating pool had shrunk! A month later, some fibroids that had started growing had also gone down in size. My diet was now on the route of the raw and wholesome (which is what R.A.W. stands for). Think of it: all uncooked food, nothing processed, no dairy, no added sugar, just things in their most natural state; raw foods. Many raw nuts and foods must be soaked first, though. I'm drinking a gallon of water or coconut water daily, unsweetened tea--not even a microwave can get near my food supply!

As my progress continues to increase, I'm just desperate for the people who are like me to embrace the benefits of a RAW lifestyle. People tend to say that a lifestyle like this is not the most sustainable. This is especially easy to appreciate when we see the unpredictable food prices see-sawing from week to week. Based on experience, I'd suggest leaving the supermarket rush! We become instead slaves to the precarious rise and fall of food prices when we don't go directly to the source--or at least as close to the farmer-source as possible. I've found such deep relief in buying instead, from our local vendors. "Does it all balance out?" you may still wonder. You'd be happy to discover that it actually does! Market-bought produce works out to be more affordable when compared to all the extra components of a meat-based dish that requires, for example, that you purchase seasonings and other add-ins to prepare the meat well, plus you actually have to purchase the meat.

If the thought of finding options that you really enjoy becomes even more daunting to you than the perceived expense of a raw-food diet, choosing and sticking to familiar fruits, vegetables, and other options until you gain more knowledge and practice can be a welcome initiation into your diet transformation. It's so important to just keep it simple at the end of the day. I can't stress enough how easy and fun it is for me just to whip together a delicious, satisfying fruit bowl after a quick chop or peel. We have such an abundance of natural resources, and I really believe that it's time we made use of them.

The resources that exist around us have the power to provide natural and holistic remedies to even severe and long-term illnesses. I have not experienced a significant flare-up of pain or any other symptoms since adopting the raw foods lifestyle. Picture yourself substituting one thing at a time: nut milk or almond milk for your typical whole milk dairy…nut cheese for your basic cheddar…fruits and dates to sweeten instead of processed sugar…I could literally go on for hours! It's possible, especially when you have people in your corner who can show you that it is working.

"Where do I get my own community?" you may then ask. Well, I seriously believe that when the time is right, many things fall into place…but then, there are times when a nudge from a person like me can help take you even a step further. I'd invite you to check out **@realplantbabe** and **@rawfoodchallengeja** or send me a message to find out more information, including how you can access coaching and a community like the awesome one that I have! I've had the pleasure of meeting such a broad spectrum of people from all walks of life who all have a quest for hope, progress partnership, and inner-to-outer renewal.

Finally, if I could leave something with you, it's that when you discover something life-changing, you can't help but share it! Go forth, eat, and live well! And remember that healing your body alone is not enough. If you are to truly transform, you must also renew your mind and spirit!

A Little Extra

*5 "Minerals from the Soil" from G. Grandma **(QUOTES)***

Now, what kind of friend would I be if I didn't share with you some of the witty wisdom "minerals" my great grandma carefully and consistently deposited in me over the years? These just might help you emotionally and spiritually too, I'm certainly learning to live better through these.

My prayer for you is that you'd learn to apply these proverbs and allow them to help guide your transformation journey:

1. **"If mi cyaa rule mi yaad, how mi fi rule mi church?"** This literally means, "If I can't earn respect and authority in my area of domain, then I won't earn it outside." This mineral from Mama, can even be applied to my personal journey now...If I can't rule my own "temple" with discipline...how can I expect to experience success in other areas of my life?

2. **"I leff yu to God."** (Usually in response to my

troublemaking/when others would engage her in arguments...) But in truth may you be granted the serenity to leave to God the things that are truly His to fix and the courage to trust that He will.

3. ***"Mi jus pray fi yu enuh...mi pray fi di whole wide world."*** Now, Mama often said in the midst of her struggles with Alzheimer's...when told who someone was/someone coming to visit...remembering/not recognizing them...-My hope is that like her your prayers will become not only for those who we love but especially for those who challenge us, it is one sound sign of maturity but more importantly spiritual wisdom.

4. ***"Yu mus forgive!"*** I can't think of another phrase that echoes Mama Freda's seemingly favorite words. I witnessed this very woman, endure a nasty one-sided conflict launched by a neighbor. She must've been the only person in our community to incite a *knocking of heads* with my great grandma...and yet, instead of

returning the favor, the very strong, very stoic Mama Freda, she cared for that woman with every ounce of kindness and love when she later fell ill. I aim, now, to be that forgiving! Forgiveness is difficult but it truly, brings FREEDOM of mind and spirit.

5. **"Share yuh husban food first."** Now, *don't get it twisted.* I'm not promoting a slavish submission that removes wifely initiative and independence. What this means to me, is that you should *prioritize* your spouse, learning how to honor and respect him. *While I'm not yet married,* these are the principles on which my relationship is built. It's a true encouragement to invest in people, in relationships and to put others above yourself.

I truly believe that if you take these lessons and apply them, you'd be the wiser--and perhaps even the kinder and more fulfilled--for it.

Conclusion

Being diagnosed with both Polycystic Ovarian Syndrome and Fibroids was one of the most dreadful days of my life. I thought my life was over; not one but two hormonal issues that were like twins from two different eggs. All along I thought I was living healthily enough. I thought I was eating the "proper way". The truth was simple but hard to swallow, I was *not* eating well. I was eating to feed diseases. I was literally eating to kill my body-not to keep it alive. Upon accepting that hard truth, I then ventured on a journey to fight back, take back control of my life *and my womanhood.*

Life is unpredictable. It often gives us a mixed bag of seeds. While we may not have a choice in the seeds handed to us, we can choose how we push for life, how we seek sunlight and water for the parts of ourselves we want to flourish and grow, yes, we can choose to bloom where we're planted. May you discover hope today. May you bloom wherever you've been planted.

Additional Resources Page

My new outlook on life has come with a transformed mental and emotional perspective. My personal motto is now:

"I persevere, "I am resilient" and "I am a risk taker."

These are known to me as my **P.R.R.** factor - the winning combination.

I know the work that I must put in. I know the journey forward is not going to be easy. I've been ashamed. I've been afraid but I know now that I must do this if I want to not only survive but *thrive!*

I've discovered a myriad of key takeaways that I'd love to share with you, so that you can equip yourselves and take the necessary steps forward.

Finally, it's important to recognize that the *symptoms of fibroids* and *PCOS* aren't just *physical.* They can creep into *every* area of our lives.

ABOUT THE AUTHOR

Stephany Staple is a dedicated farmer, PCOS, and fibroid advocate. She hails from a small town in Clarendon, Jamaica. Stephany is passionate about life and staying healthy. She has dedicated the last three years to research and personal experience to understand the critical connection between diet, health, and vitality. Her background in agriculture equips her with key knowledge of growing food, vital in taking charge of her health.

With genuine warmth and a sprinkle of humor, she is committed to fostering a community of support and providing tools for others to reclaim health, discover inner strength, and flourish in all aspects of life.

"The Good Seed" is her first book and is dedicated to her great-grandmother, who was instrumental in her upbringing.

SOCIAL PAGES ON INSTAGRAM

@stephany_staple

@r.a.w.e.a.t.s

@realplantbabe

@rawfoodchallengeja

@iseeedyouths

Please Follow, Like and Share.

Thank You for Reading!